Alzheimer

The disease and the care

Causes, symptoms and prevention
through healthy living

By Claire .C. Philip

Copyright

Disclaimer

Table of Content

Chapter 1

Introduction

Alzheimer's disease

Alzheimer's disease is known to be the most common type of dementia. It is a neurodegenerative disease in which the death of brain cells causes memory loss and cognitive decline. It accounts for 60 to 80 percent of cases of dementia in the United States.

The human brain is made up of billions of nerve cells that are connected. Alzheimer disease occurs when plaques containing beta-amyloid develop in the brain, thereby cutting off the connections between the cells. It is a deposit of protein in the brain which forms abnormal structures called 'plaques' and 'tangles.' Initially, symptoms are hardly noticed but become severe over time. The symptoms worsen, and it becomes difficult for the person involves to remember recent events, to reason and to identify people they know.

Alzheimer disease is a continuous decline in thinking, behavioral, and social skills that interrupts a person's ability to function independently.

Finally, a person with Alzheimer's disease probably needs full-time assistance.

Although the actual cause of Alzheimer disease is not yet ascertained, some things are thought to increase the risk of developing the condition. They include:

Aging

A family history of the condition

Untreated depression

Lifestyle factors

Chapter 2

Severity types of Alzheimer

Almost everyone with Alzheimer's disease will finally arrive at the same symptoms, which include memory loss, confusion, trouble with once-familiar tasks, hallucination, and making decisions. Although the effects of the disease are similar, it is classified in different ways. A patient may experience any or all number of the symptoms that mark each stage

Mild Alzheimer's

This includes the onset of cognitive impairment that causes difficulties in recalling daily routine such as tasks at work, paying bills, and others. These changes in a person's abilities or behavior may only be minor. These symptoms may not be noticed as a sign of AD, and they are not very serious, the patients at this stage with a certain amount of difficulty manage to remain functional. They take a longer time to perform the same task which they used to do quicker before, and this becomes a pattern. It may not be noticeable to others, except family members and close friends.

Common symptoms of Mild Stage Alzheimer

- o Slight memory loss in terms of forgetting what has just been read, losing items, and repeating questions
- o Difficulty in remembering some names or words
- o Mood swings, including sessions of depression, anxiety, apathy, irritability, and apathy. These symptoms can result in personality change, like becoming withdrawn or lacking motivation.
- o Confusion and disorientation
- o Trouble learning new ideas, and a lack of desire to try new things
- o The trouble with steady concentration, such as losing the train of thought in mid-sentence or quickly loss of interest in an activity.
- o Slow in speech.
- o Always allow the patient to maintain independence and be active because it helps prevent anxiety and depression.

Moderate Alzheimer's

Here the symptoms of moderate Alzheimer's are more intense because of a significant amount of neuronal damage. This stage is the longest stage, and a patient may remain in it for many years before the condition significantly advances. They become increasingly dependent on others and often begin to need more help with day-to-day life and self-care. This may lead to anger and frustration in patients and can result in them reacting in unpredicted ways. Due to the amount of memory loss, the confusion becomes worse. These individuals, though physically agile, as the delusions take over the sensory processing of their thoughts, are not able to perform routine tasks. This individual will experience most of the symptoms that occur in the mild stages but with a growing degree of severity.

For instance

- o Memory loss may now span to a person forgetting his or her own personal history, personal details such as a home address, telephone number, and increase in nervousness that can cause the person to wander.

- o There is an increase in confusion and disorientation, resulting in losing track of dates, seasons, and passage of time. Extra care is unavoidable needed in this case to help with dressing in clothes appropriate to the time of day and the season.
- o The individual is always reminded to eat, groom, bathe, and use the bathroom. In some case, the individuals may find it difficult controlling their bladder and bowel movements.
- o This stage always comes with hallucinations (seeing things that are not there) or delusions (believing things that aren't true) experience, which sometimes leads to paranoia and aggressive behavior toward caregivers and loved ones.
- o There is an increase in difficulty with speech, which can lead to forgetting words, incoherent with sounding of words or making up new words.
- o The person is not getting enough sleep.

- o Continuous change in mood, like depression, confusion, anxiety, anger, and frustration, are inevitable.

Severe Alzheimer's/Late Stage

At this stage, the brain cell starts dying due to spreading of plaques and tangles, which results in shrinkage of brain tissue. The individuals at this stage are typically bedridden and are hardly able to communicate. They required constant supervision and frequent professional care.

Symptoms of Moderate Alzheimer

- o Confusion will set in, and the persons become unaware of their environment and surroundings.
- o The person finds it difficult to recognize faces of closest friends and relatives.
- o Remembering most details of personal history becomes a thing of the past.
- o The persons find it difficult to control the bladder and bowel movement at all times.
- o Changes in major personality and potential behavior problems will increase drastically.
- o The person begins to wander continuously.

- o   This stage requires assistance with activities of daily living such as toileting and bathing.

As the diseases progress, the person involve loses the ability to communicate or respond to their environment. Some may still be able to utter words and phrases; they have no insight into their condition and will always need assistance with all activities of daily living. In the final stages of Alzheimer's, the probability that the person may lose the ability to swallow is high.

How to cope with the late stage of Alzheimer's disease

Caregiving becomes harder when a person moves to the last stage of Alzheimer disease. At this stage, you are required to make a decision on whether to manage your loved one's condition at home or take them to a skilled care facility or hospice. You aim now as a caregiver should focus on preserving quality and dignity of life. Typically a person in the late stage of Alzheimer's disease loses the ability to express needs and talk, although some core of the person's self may remain. This means that the caregiver may continue to connect with the person throughout the late stage of the disease.

There are many good ways to give quality care regardless of where the care takes place; the endpoint is making sure the person receives the care needed.

The person suffering from Alzheimer disease at this point experiences the world through senses. Caregivers are encouraged to express their caring through touch, sight, sound, taste, and smell. Examples are

- o   Playing the patients favorite music
- o   Reading parts of books that have meaning for the person
- o   Looking and focusing on old photos together
- o   Preparing the persons favorite food
- o   Rubbing lotion with a favorite scent into the skin
- o   Brushing the person's hair
- o   Sitting and relaxing outside together on a nice day

Roles of Caregivers

1) Feeding

As Alzheimer's disease progresses to the last stage, many people lose interest in food.

Monitoring the person eating habit is one of the most important daily caregiving tasks. As a person becomes less active, less food is required. Importantly a person in this stage of the disease also may lose appetite or forget to eat. Adding a little sugar to food and serving favorite foods may encourage eating. Try to serve meals in a quiet environment. Another good option for food is finger foods and protein milkshakes. Encourage self-feeding, slowly offer food and drink and alternating bites of food with something to drink (fluids). Choose soft food that can be chew and swallow easily. You are encouraged to thicken liquids as the person develops problems swallowing foods. If weight loss is observed, the doctor may suggest taking supplements between meals to add calories.

To help with the digestion, keep the person upright for thirty minutes after eating and allow plenty of time for eating.

2) Swallowing Problems and precautions

The progression of Alzheimer disease to the late stage is a serious problem because chewing and swallowing become difficult for the person. It is likely that the person might choke on a bite of food and the probability of the food going into the lungs is high, which can cause pneumonia.

The following are swallowing guideline.

- o The prepared food should be tender and cut into pieces.
- o Grind food or make it liquid by using a blender or baby food grinder.
- o Provide tender/soft foods, in the likes of as ice cream, milkshakes, soups, yogurt, applesauce, custard, and gelatin.
- o Avoid the use of a straw because it may cause more swallowing problems. Taking a small sip from a cup is preferable.
- o Observe the quantity of milk consumed by the person, if it tends to catch in the throat, reduce the consumption quantity.
- o Cold drinks are easier to swallow, so give the person more cold drinks.
- o Avoid giving the person thin liquids like coffee, water, tea, or broth, because they are the most difficult to swallow. You can buy Thick-It® at

most pharmacies and add it to liquid to make them thicker. Another alternative to thicken liquid is using ice cream and sherbet.

o   Give the person time to chew and swallow each food properly before taking another bite. Do not be in a hurry.

o   Avoid feeding a drowsy person or a person lying down. Make sure the person is in an upright sitting position during a meal and stays upright for at least 20 minutes after the meal.

o   Make sure you position the person neck forward and the chin down when swallowing.

o   Gently Stroke the person's neck in a downward motion and say "swallow" to remind the person to swallow.

o   Make the eating area quiet by turning off gadgets like TV, CD player, or radio that might cause distraction.

o   Let the mealtime be the same each day.

o   Use a colorful and attractive plate to serve a meal so that the person can see the food.

o   Find out from the doctor if the person's medicine can be crushed or taken in liquid form.

Helping an Alzheimer patient to eat at this last stage is a very tedious task. But you can make it easier by planning ahead and having the food ready.

3) Bowel and bladder function

Difficulty with using the restroom (toileting) is very common at this stage in the disease. The person may need assistance to walk to the restroom and helped through the process. During late Alzheimer, disease incontinence is also common.

To maintain bowel and bladder function:

o   **Set a toileting schedule.** Keep a written note of when the person enters the bathroom, and when and how much the person eats and drinks. This will help you make a plan of the person's natural routine, and then you can plan a schedule. If the person is not able to get to the toilet, use disposable adult briefs and bed pads.

o   **Limit liquids before bedtime.** Limit the liquid before bedtime but do not eliminate liquids at least two hours before bedtime. Make sure to provide adequate fluids for the person all through the day to avoid dehydration.

o **Monitor bowel movements**. Bowel movement does not happen every day, but if you observe that there was no bowel movement for three consecutive days, know that constipation has set in. In this situation, you can add natural laxatives to the diet, such as prunes or fiber-rich foods (bran or whole-grain bread). If constipation continues, consult your doctor.

4) **Body and Skin Health.**

A Person with late-stage of Alzheimer's can become either bedridden or chair- bound. The lack of ability to move around can cause pressure sores, skin breakdown, and freezing of joints as the case may be.

A physical therapist is needed to show the caregiver (you) how to transfer the person safely, change person position in bed, and do some range-of-motion exercises to prevent pressure sores and stiffness. You are to learn special skills to keep you from hurting yourself when moving the person.

5) How to move or lift the person

o   Bend at the knees and straighten up by using your thigh muscles, not your back.

o   Straighten your back and don't bend at the waist.

o   Hold the person as close to avoid reaching away from your body.

o   Place one of your foot in front of the other, or open your feet comfortably apart for a wide base of support.

o   Use a little step to move the person from one seat to another. Don't twist your body

o   Getting equipment like a transfer belt or a lift will help to make the task easier. To move using transfer belt: wrap the belt around the person's waist and slide the person to the edge of the chair or bed, face the person, place your hands on each side of the person's waist. After that, bend your knees and pull up using your thigh muscles to bring up the person from a seated to a standing position.

o   For the person's comfort, it is advisable to use wedge-shaped cushions and a special mattress.

The equipment will help to prevent pressure
sores and aid in moving the person every two
hours.

6) **How to keep an Alzheimer patient's skin and body healthy:**

o Change the person's position at least every two
hours to improve blood circulation and relieve
body pressure. Use pillows to support arms and
legs and make sure the person is properly
aligned and comfortable.

o How to lift properly and turn the person
without causing harm or injury should be taught
by a care provider or physical therapist. Avoid
lifting by pulling on the person's arm or
shoulders.

o It is very important to keep the persons skin
clean and dry. Use very gentle motions during
cleaning and avoid friction to prevent skin from
easy tear and bruise. Bath or wash the body with
mild soap and blot dry. Check for rashes, sores,
or breakdown daily.

o Use pillows or pads to protect the joints like
elbows, heels, hips, and other bony areas. If you

use a skin moisturizer on these areas, gently apply it, and avoid massaging it.

o Joint freezing happens when a person is confined to a particular chair or bed. It is advisable to engage in an in range-of-motion exercise in order to prevent the freezing of the joint. This exercise is all about moving the arms and legs two or three times a day after bathing whiles, the skin and muscles are still warm. During this range of motion exercises, hold the person's arms or legs, one at a time, and move and bend it several times a day. The exercise helps to prevent stiffness of the arms, legs, and hands. It also prevents pressure or bedsores.

Always consult your doctor before starting any form of exercise for a patient living with Alzheimer disease.

7) Dental, Skin, and Foot Problems

Dental, skin, and foot problems mostly happen during the late stage of Alzheimer's disease. The lack of ability to move around during late-stage Alzheimer's disease can make a person more exposed to infections.

8) How to prevent mouth and teeth infections:

o Practicing good oral hygiene bring to a minimum the risk of bacteria in the mouth which can lead to pneumonia. Always brush the person's teeth after each meal. If the person is putting on dentures, remove and clean them every night. Use a good soft toothbrush or moistened gauze pad to clean the gums, tongue, and other soft mouth tissues.

o If you notice any cut, clean and treat immediately with warm soapy water and apply an antibiotic ointment, seek professional medical help if the cut is deep.

o Protect the person against flu and pneumonia. The flu (influenza) can lead to pneumonia (infection in the lungs). It's important for the person with Alzheimer's as well as the caregivers to get flu vaccines every year to help decrease the risk. A vaccine is available every five years to guard against pneumococcal pneumonia (a severe lung infection caused by bacteria).

9) Pain and illness

In the late stage of Alzheimer pain, communicating with people becomes difficult. Consult a doctor as soon as possible if you suspect pain or illness try to find the likely cause. Pain medication may be prescribed in some cases.

How to recognize pain and illness:

There are physical signs you can look out for which includes pale skin tone; dry, flushed skin tone; pale gums; vomiting, mouth sores, feverish skin; or swelling of any part of the body.

Always be attentive to nonverbal sign. Gestures, spoken sounds, and facial expressions (wincing, for example) may be a sign of pain or discomfort.

Be observant to changes in behavior like agitation, anxiety, trembling, shouting, and sleeping problems can also be signs of pain.

10) Skin problems in the late stage of Alzheimer

Skin problems or pressure sores occur when the person stops walking or stays in one position for too long.

How to prevent skin or pressure sores

- o If the person is in a sitting position, move at least every 2 hours.
- o If the person is lying down, move the person at least every hour.
- o Place a 4-inch foam pad on top of the person's mattress.
- o Check the foam pad and make sure that it is comfortable for the person.
- o Some persons are allergic to the foam pad, and some find these pads too hot for sleeping. If the foam pad is a problem, you can substitute and get pads filled with gel, water, or water.
- o Adjust and position the person to sink a little when lying down on the pad. Also, the pad should fit securely around the body.

How to check for pressure sores:

- o Check if you will notice redness or sores on the person's heels, buttocks, hips, shoulders, back, and elbows.

- o Seek the doctor advice on what to do if you noticed pressure sores. Try to keep the person off the affected area.
- o Here is what to do to help take care of the feet of Alzheimer patients, if they were unable to do that.
- o Soak the person's feet in warm water; use a mild soap to wash the feet and look for cuts, corns, and calluses.
- o After washing the feet, put lotion on the feet to prevent the skin from becoming dry and cracked.
- o Cut or file their toenails.

If you notice a case of diabetes or sores on the feet, inform a foot doctor or a podiatrist at once.

11) Body Jerking

Myoclonus is a condition that from time to time happens with Alzheimer's. It looks more like a seizure, but the person will not pass out. The person's arms, legs, or whole-body may jerk. Tell the doctor immediately if you observe these signs. The doctor may prescribe one or more medicines to help reduce the symptoms.

Chapter 3

Onset or Trigger type Alzheimer

Early-Onset Alzheimer's

Early-onset of Alzheimer is a rare form of dementia that affects people below 65 years of age. This condition is sporadic, and of all the people who have Alzheimer's disease, about 5 out of 100 develop symptoms between their late 40s or early 50s.

 Early-onset Alzheimer's disease has closely the same symptoms with those of other forms of Alzheimer's disease.

Alzheimer Early-onset symptoms

- o Forgetting newly learned information or important dates
- o They keep asking for the same piece of information over and over again.
- o Find it challenging to solve fundamental problems, such as keeping track of bills or following a favorite recipe.
- o Forgetting dates or time of year

- o Losing track of where you are and how you got there
- o The person will have trouble with depth perception or other vision problems.
- o Difficulty fitting in conversations or finding the right word for something
- o Misplacing of things and not being able to retrace your steps to find it
- o Increase in poor judgment
- o Withdrawal from work and social situations
- o They will a lot of mood Changes and personality

Types of early onset of Alzheimer

1) Common Alzheimer Disease

Most people with early-onset Alzheimer's disease have the common form of Alzheimer's disease. For older people with Alzheimer disease, the condition will progress in roughly the same way.

2) Genetic Alzheimer's disease.

This is an extremely rare case. A few hundred people have genes that directly contribute to Alzheimer's disease called familial Alzheimer disease. These groups of people begin showing symptoms of the disease in their 30s, 40s, or 50s.

They may have a parent or grandparent who also developed Alzheimer's at a younger age.

Distinct features of this condition are considered the outcome of a defect in Chromosome 14.

Early-onset Alzheimer's that runs in families is connected to these three genes

 APP genes

PSEN 1 genes

PSEN 2 genes

These genes differ from the APOE gene that can increase your risk of Alzheimer's in general.

These three genes brought together account for less than 1 percent of all Alzheimer's disease cases but about 60 to 70 percent of early-onset Alzheimer's cases. You may develop Alzheimer before the age of 65 if you have a genetic mutation in one of those three genes.

There is the availability of genetic testing for these mutations but first, go for genetic counseling to examine the pros and cons before the test. The early detection of the disease is important in preventing or slowing down its progression.

If you have early-onset Alzheimer's connected to one of the three genes or carry any form of these genes without symptoms. Now is time to talk to your doctor about taking part in a research study. With this study, researchers hope to learn more about the causes and progression of the disease and find new treatments.

Accurate diagnosis is critical

To rule out other potential issues and get the most suitable treatment for personal and professional reasons, an accurate diagnosis of early-onset Alzheimer's is vital. A doctor will then make a diagnosis of Alzheimer's disease with a few tests.

First, the doctor will ask of a medical history of the patient and also perform some cognitive tests of memory, problem-solving, and other mental skills.

Secondly, the doctor may also test the blood, urine, and spinal fluid of the patient.

Finally, CT and MRI scans of the brain can give the doctor a run down and a closer look at the brain tissue to disclose the extent of the damage.

This diagnosis is fundamental steps in helping the family respond with the best understanding and compassion.

The diagnosis gives you and your family more time to make important decisions about financial and legal issues.

Another advantage of early diagnosis is that it allows you to explain your condition to your employer at work, for a more convenient schedule or better still a lighter workload.

Coping with early onset of Alzheimer

People diagnosis with early-onset Alzheimer's disease may face some unique challenges.

Learning about the unique challenges of living with early-onset is the first step in understanding the effect the disease will have on you and your family. It can help dismiss some of the anxieties and fears you may have about the future and give you enough time to focus on the things that bring you joy.

Some common issues associated with early-onset Alzheimer are:

a. Dealing with stigmas and stereotypes about the disease, which can have a significant influence on your well-being and quality of life. Stigma brings about withdrawal and isolation from a relationship. You don't need to fear stigma instead fight it.

b. People find it difficult to believe they have the disease or question the diagnosis due to their young age.

c. People with early-onset Alzheimer's has a high risk of losing their relationships or jobs; instead, as a result of this misunderstanding rather than being recognized as medically ill or disabled.

d. It may also result in loss of income from being diagnosed while still working.

Now that the disease is still in its early stages, it's necessary to think about the future, which includes:

planning financially ahead to put critical financial and legal plan in place. Working with employers on present and potential job responsibilities, updating and clarifying health insurance coverage, and getting all important documents ready to avoid to be taken unaware should your health take a turn for the worse.

Tips on how to cope with early onset of Alzheimer for couples

A diagnosis of early-onset Alzheimer's disease doesn't just affect those with the disease. After the diagnosis, spouses or partners often feel a sense of loneliness or loss as they are faced with spending many years without an active partner.

- o The most difficult aspect of it is losing the romantic part of the relationship. Also changing to a caregiver status tends to complicate the relationship.

- o The couple should talk about what kind of help they need from each other. The affected spouse should communicate about changes they are experiencing and ways in which their needs also may have changed. Always be courageous and ask for help.

- o Go ahead and participate in as many activities with your partner that you presently enjoy and adjust where necessary. Alternatively, look for new activities that you can enjoy together.
- o Have a folder of resources you may need available as the disease progresses.
- o Register with Alzheimer support group or find an available counselor who works with couples facing issues you feel challenged by, such altering roles in the relationship and sexuality.

Ways and how to let the kids know

It is quite painful to know that family dynamics will change in a matter of time. The parental role will also change.

It may be difficult for children to understand the early onset of Alzheimer disease diagnosis. Discuss with your partner know the type of information your child can comprehend and how much he or she can cope with.

Some children may end up blaming themselves, become angry, or react in many numbers of ways. It is also common to think about the role you will play in the significant events of your children's lives as they grow older, and as the disease advances.

To reduce the effect on the children:

- Find activities you can enjoy together and participate actively.
- Let your children know what you are experiencing and honestly talk with them.
- Find a registered support group for children, and go with your kids to some of your counseling sessions. Inform your child's school counselor and social worker about your condition.
- Try and keep a written note, audio record or video of your thoughts, feelings, and experiences for your children. They'll appreciate your sharing your wisdom and memories.

One Challenging aspect of early diagnosis is coping with your emotions. One of the best ways you can help your child overcome the challenges of living with the disease is to take good care of your physical and emotional needs.

Financial issues

All most all the people with early-onset Alzheimer's often have to stop work, and this lead to a loss of income which is a major concern.

It might get worse if spouses or partners also quit their jobs to become full-time caregivers.

Getting Ready for the Future?

There are many plans you can make now that will be a big help later. For example, Try and see a lawyer to know the type of arrangements you'll need. Give someone "power of attorney," to lets the people you love make health and money decisions for you when it will be difficult to do that on your own.

You also need to plan how you'll pay for some of your future health costs. Some of the things to consider are safety equipment you'll need at home or getting help from a professional or registered caregiver. If possible, engage your family, talk about your finance, and how much money you're likely to need to get proper care when you can no longer do that on your own.

The important thing is to realize what you want, make a precise, realistic plan, and inform your loved ones.

Healthy living

Yes, Alzheimer's disease has no cure presently; you can make the best of this disorder, focusing on a combination of social, mental, and physically stimulating activities. These include:

Keep an active mind

To keep an active mind, you must inculcate these listed activities in your life activities to help form the vital neural connection that can last for a lifetime.

- o The stimulating activities may shield people from cognitive decline and also has the advantage of an increase in social interactions with family and friends.
- o Reading more challenging books progressively
- o Learning how to use a musical instrument
- o Studying a new language

o   Creating art

o   Playing chess, crossword puzzles, brain teaser

o   Engaging in other mental activities like
    conversing and singing

o   Reading newspapers, magazine, and journals.

o   Exercising Regularly

o   Regularly exercise is vital because it improves
    overall physical, mental fitness, and emotional
    health. It also increases blood circulation in the
    brain. Exercises help in Releasing stress,
    maintaining a healthy weight, and an increase in
    flexibility.

o   Aerobic exercise, strength training, and activity
    to increase flexibility are a good combination
    and highly recommended.

People living with Alzheimer disease can participate in any of these physical exercises depending on the stage of the disease and also with accommodations.

There are some suggested exercises put in place for people living with Alzheimer disease.

o   Walking that is accompanied by a companion

o   Register in aerobic exercise classes at a center for seniors or local swimming pool.

o   The person should participate in light gardening.

o   Modified sports games with love ones

It is still worthwhile to have an outlet for physical activities as the disease progresses in order to maintain muscle tone, elevate mood, and physical strength. Inform your health care provider before you engage in any form of exercise so that a suitable exercise program will be tailored for your specific need.

Healthy eating

Eating healthy foods is the right step to stay well.

Eating a Mediterranean diet that is rich in whole grain, fruits, vegetables, olive oil, fish, moderate amounts of poultry, eggs, dairy, and low fats, and sugar can minimize the risk of many chronic diseases.

Give the persons varieties about what to eat and make sure that you buy foods the person likes and can eat. Keeping to familiar routines and serving favorite foods can make mealtimes easier for Alzheimer patients. They can help the person know what to expect and feel more comfortable. The family should not forget to tell the home health aide or other professional providers care about the person's preferences.

Treatment

Early-onset Alzheimer's disease currently has no cure, but it is important to manage your condition by staying as positive as you can. Try different ways to relax like deep breathing or yoga and keep up with the activities you still enjoy. They are some medications that help people with early onset of Alzheimer maintain mental function, control behavior, and slow the progression of the disease such as

 donepezil (Aricept), rivastigmine (Exelon), galantamine (Razadyne), and memantine (Namenda).

These drugs are known to delay or improve your symptoms for a few months to a few years. They may give you more time to live independently.

NOTE: DO NOT TAKE ANY MEDICATION WITHOUT YOUR DOCTOR PRESCRIPTION

Some health tips for managing the person living with Alzheimer diseases.

- o See mealtimes as opportunities for social interaction. Always display a warm and happy tone of voice when talking with a person living with Alzheimer disease.
- o It helps with the mood.
- o Be patient and give the person plenty of time to finish the meal.
- o Respect the personal, cultural, and religious food favorites, such as eating tortillas as aa alternative for bread or avoiding pork.
- o Do not alter the person meal time; continue to serve meals at those times.
- o If possible, serve meals in a consistent, familiar place and way.
- o Avoid new routines like serving breakfast to a person who has never routinely eaten breakfast.

Late-onset Alzheimer

Late Alzheimer is the most common form of dementia disease, and it affects people older than 65 years of age. It may or may not be a genetic trigger. So far, researchers are unable to find a particular gene that triggers it, and further research is going on. No one knows for sure why some people get it, and others don't. A recent finding shows that estimates of 5.7 million Americans are living with Alzheimer disease-related dementia. The number of individuals affected is growing rapidly because of an aging population.

Symptoms of late-onset Alzheimer

- o Vascular risk factor, Sleep disorders
- o Behavior changes and severe mood swings.
- o In-depth of confusion about time, place, and life events
- o Suspicions about family, friends, or caregivers
- o Difficulty speaking, swallowing or walking
- o Severe memory loss

Chapter 3

Who is at risk?

There is not a single cause of Alzheimer's disease say, researchers. The disease might come from multiple factors, such as genetics, lifestyle, and environment.

Some of the factors identified by scientists that increase the risk of Alzheimer disease are age, family history, and heredity. Other factors include head injury, heart head connection,

1) **Age**

Age is one of the most significant known risk factors for Alzheimer. Alzheimer disease is not a normal part of aging.

Most people living with the disease are 65 years upward. The risk of Alzheimer's doubles every five years after 65 years of age. The risk reaches almost one-third after 85 years of age.

2) **Family History**

If more than one family member has the illness, the risk of Alzheimer disease increases which may be a result of heredity or environmental factor.

3) Genetics (heredity)

Genes play a significant role in Alzheimer says the scientists. Alzheimer genes have been found in two categories of genes that stimulate whether a person develops a disease. Those genes are risk genes and deterministic genes. The study has it that deterministic genes cause less than 1 percent of Alzheimer cases.

4) **Lifestyle**

It is vital to live a healthy lifestyle, especially from mid-life onwards, and the risk of developing Alzheimer disease will decrease.

A healthy lifestyle comes to inform of eating a healthy balanced diet, regular physical exercise, and keeping to a healthy weight.

5) **Head injury**

Always protect your brain by wearing a helmet, buckling your seat belt when participating in sports to avoid head injury. People who experience severe or repeated head injuries have a high risk of developing dementia. The onset of dementia may be linked to deposits that form in the brain as a result of an injury.

Other factors like a high level of cholesterol and blood pressure may also increase the risk of Alzheimer disease

Chapter 4

Prevention

How can the risk be reduced?

Alzheimer disease can be reduced by living a healthy life.

Activities needed to maintain or improve brain health.

- o   Be physically active and exercise regularly.
- o   Always eat a well-balanced diet that is rich in fruits, cereals, legumes, fish, and vegetables.
- o   Detest from smoking and excessive alcohol intake.
- o   Monitor your numbers and keep blood pressure, cholesterol, and blood sugar at a healthy level.
- o   Maintain body weight within recommended ranges.
- o   Stay connected with family and friends, and regularly interact with others.
- o   Reduce stress and treat depression.

- o Keep your mind and brain active by trying something new, for example, learning a new language or playing games.
- o Control the onset of type 2 diabetes.
- o Always protect your head when you are engaged in sporting activities by wearing a helmet.
- o Always make sure that you have enough sleep.

Care at the end of life

Many patients with a neurological disorder can't think clearly or articulate their wishes for end-of-life care.

When a person with late-stage Alzheimer's nears the end of life and has lost the capacity to make medical decisions. The families must make choices on the person's behalf. The healthcare provider should engage family early on in advance care planning by asking whether the patient has put in place advance directives that specify his or her wishes. If there are no such directives, the families must put in their best choice based on what they believe the person would want. All end-of-life decisions made by the family should respect the person's values and wishes. The decisions should also maintain the person comfort and dignity. The

Alzheimer's Association® is always ready to help you prepare for making end-of-life decisions.

There are some necessary things you'll need to consider.

- o Talk regularly to your loved one's primary doctor and make sure you understand the medical care plan.
- o Get their financial plans in order and will too.
- o Decide the place of death, whether at home, hospital, or nursing home.
- o Find out if your insurance cover hospice, palliative care, and other services available in your area. If it does, decide what palliative care or hospice team, you will need their assistance. Make sure they are Medicare certified.
- o Write their obituary.
- o Decide which funeral home you'll use a cemetery or a burial plot and what the funeral plans will be.